LOW FODMAP DIET COOKBOOK FOR BEGINNERS

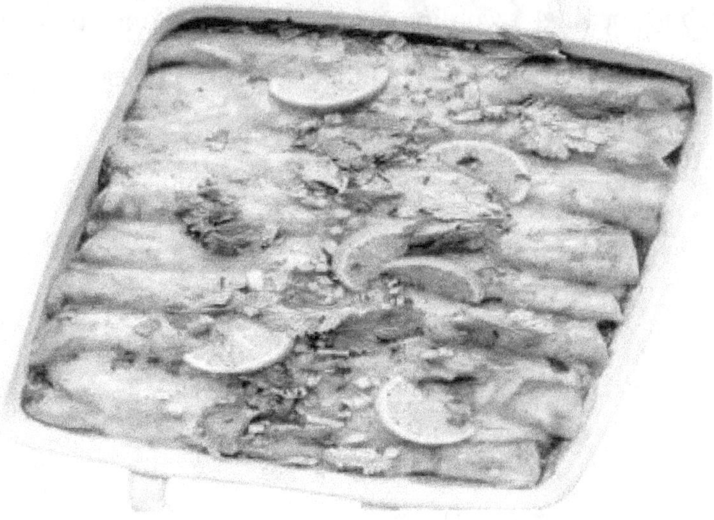

Simple And Delicious Recipes To Take Control Of IBS And Other Digestive Disorders. Includes 30 Days Meal Plan

Katherine J. Filer

Copyright 2023, Katherine J. Filer

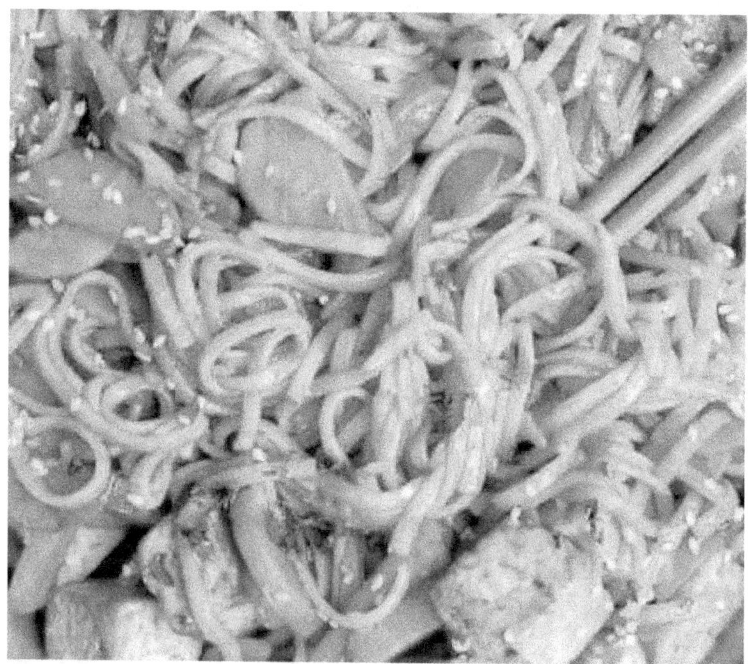

Table of Contents

INTRODUCTION

In the gentle twilight of a bustling city, Patricia found herself entrenched in a relentless battle against digestive discomfort. A young professional navigating the whirlwind of a demanding career, she grappled with mysterious gut issues that sapped her energy and overshadowed her days with an unwelcome heaviness. Countless doctor visits and conflicting advice left her feeling adrift, until a chance encounter with a nutritionist transformed her life.

As Patricia delved into the world of nutrition, she unearthed the transformative power of the Low FODMAP Diet. What initially seemed like a mere list of food choices became a beacon of hope and restoration. Gradually, as she embraced this dietary approach, relief cascaded over her, the once burdensome symptoms began to wane, offering her a renewed sense of vitality and joy.

The story of Patricia is not an isolated tale; it's a testament to the potential held within the pages of this guide. Welcome to the "Low FODMAP Diet Cookbook for Beginners." Here, within these pages, lies a treasure full of not just recipes, but a holistic approach to using food as medicine.

Imagine savoring delicious meals that not only tantalize the taste buds but also nurture your body from within. Consider the profound impact of understanding how the food on your plate can be a potent ally in combating and preventing digestive distress and related health concerns. This isn't merely a cookbook; it's a guide to redefining your relationship with food and harnessing its incredible healing potential.

As you embark on this journey, allow yourself to be captivated by the synergy of flavors and the profound impact of nutrition on your wellbeing. Join us in unlocking the doors to a vibrant and fulfilling life through the gateway of the Low FODMAP Diet. Together, let's embrace this transformative approach to eating, paving the way for a healthier, more invigorated you.

CHAPTER 1

Understanding the Low FODMAP Diet

What are FODMAPs?

FODMAPs stand for Fermentable Oligosaccharides, Disaccharides, Monosaccharides, and Polyols. They are a group of short-chain carbohydrates and sugar alcohols found in various foods.

These compounds are known for their ability to ferment in the gut, drawing in water and producing gas as they undergo fermentation. For some individuals, especially those with sensitive digestive systems or certain gastrointestinal conditions like irritable bowel syndrome (IBS), these FODMAPs can trigger symptoms such as bloating, gas, abdominal pain, diarrhea, or constipation.

Examples of foods high in FODMAPs include certain fruits (like apples, cherries, and watermelon), certain vegetables (such as onions, garlic, and asparagus), certain grains (like wheat and rye), and dairy products containing lactose, and sweeteners like honey and certain artificial sweeteners.

The low FODMAP diet involves restricting or reducing the intake of these fermentable carbohydrates to alleviate gastrointestinal symptoms and improve digestive health. This dietary approach can vary in its specifics and is often personalized based on individual tolerances and sensitivities to different FODMAP groups.

How FODMAPS Affect Digestive Health

FODMAPs can affect digestive health in several ways. When these fermentable carbohydrates and sugar alcohols are consumed and reach the small intestine, they can cause issues for some individuals:

1. Fermentation and Gas Production: FODMAPs are fermentable, which means gut bacteria break them down, producing gases like hydrogen, methane, and carbon dioxide. This fermentation process can lead to bloating, abdominal distension, and discomfort due to the increased gas production in the intestines.

2. Osmotic Effects: FODMAPs draw water into the intestines due to their osmotic properties. This influx of water can contribute to diarrhea or changes in bowel habits for some people.

3. Disturbance in Gut Motility: FODMAPs may alter the movement of the intestines, leading to either increased or decreased motility. This disturbance can result in symptoms like constipation or diarrhea, depending on the individual's reaction to specific FODMAPs.

4. Interaction with Gut Sensitivity: For individuals with a sensitive gut or underlying conditions like IBS, FODMAPs can trigger pain receptors in the intestines, leading to discomfort, cramping, and pain.

Overall, the impact of FODMAPs on digestive health varies among individuals. Some people are more sensitive to certain types of FODMAPs than others. Following a low-FODMAP diet may help alleviate these symptoms by reducing the intake of these fermentable carbohydrates and thus minimizing the distress they cause in the digestive system.

Benefits of Adopting a Low-FODMAP Diet

Adopting a low-FODMAP diet can offer several benefits, especially for individuals with sensitive digestive systems or specific gastrointestinal conditions like irritable bowel syndrome (IBS). Here are ten benefits of following a low-FODMAP diet:

1. Reduced Digestive Symptoms: By avoiding high-FODMAP foods, individuals often experience a decrease in symptoms like bloating, gas, abdominal pain, diarrhea, and constipation, providing relief from discomfort associated with these digestive issues.

2. Improved Quality of Life: Minimizing or eliminating distressing gastrointestinal symptoms can significantly enhance one's overall wellbeing, leading to a better quality of life and improved daily functioning.

3. Identification of Trigger Foods: Following a low-FODMAP diet involves a structured elimination and reintroduction process, helping individuals identify specific foods that trigger their digestive symptoms, allowing for a personalized approach to managing their diet.

4. Better Bowel Regularity: For those experiencing irregular bowel habits, such as alternating constipation and diarrhea, adhering to a low-FODMAP diet can help regulate bowel movements and promote more consistent and predictable patterns.

5. Enhanced Nutrient Absorption: By reducing gut inflammation and improving digestive comfort, a low-FODMAP diet can optimize nutrient absorption, ensuring the body absorbs essential vitamins, minerals, and other nutrients more effectively.

6. Balanced Gut Micro biota: While the low-FODMAP diet limits certain fermentable carbohydrates, it doesn't eliminate them entirely. Over time, this approach can support a more balanced and diverse gut micro biota, which is crucial for overall gut health.

7. Potential Weight Management: Some individuals may find that a low-FODMAP diet aids in weight management due to reduced bloating and discomfort, potentially leading to healthier eating habits and more mindful food choices.

8. Relief from Chronic Conditions: For people with chronic gastrointestinal disorders like IBS or inflammatory bowel diseases, adopting a low-FODMAP diet might offer significant relief and better disease management.

9. Improved Energy Levels: Minimizing digestive discomfort often results in increased energy levels and decreased fatigue, allowing individuals to engage in daily activities more comfortably and with vitality.

10. Better Psychological Wellbeing: Relief from digestive distress can positively impact mental health, reducing stress, anxiety, and the emotional burden often associated with gastrointestinal symptoms.

It's important to note that while a low-FODMAP diet can offer these benefits, it's advisable to undertake this dietary approach under the guidance of a healthcare professional or a registered dietitian to ensure proper nutritional balance and personalized guidance throughout the process.

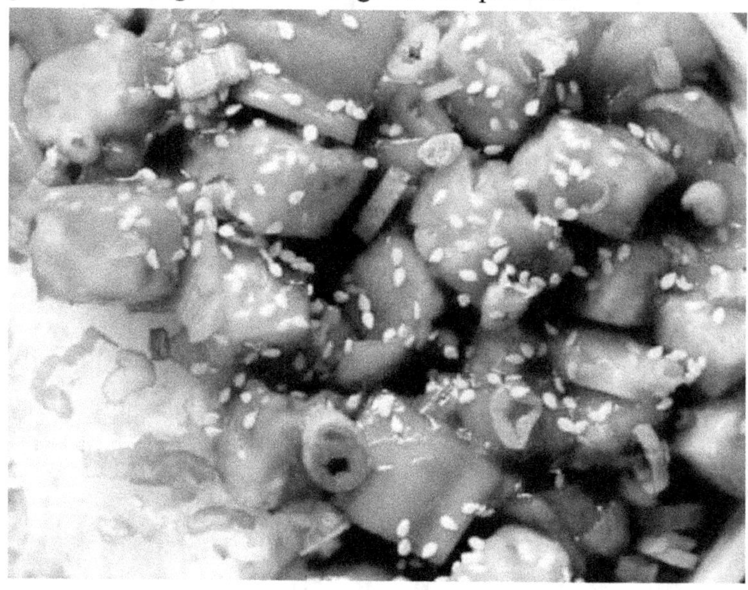

CHAPTER 2

Getting Started with the Low-FODMAP Diet

THE BASICS OF LOW-FODMAP EATING

Identifying High And Low FODMAP Foods

Identifying high and low FODMAP foods is a crucial aspect of following a low-FODMAP diet. Here's a breakdown of how these foods are categorized:

High-FODMAP Foods:

1. Oligosaccharides: Examples include wheat, rye, onions, garlic, and legumes (like chickpeas and lentils).

2. Disaccharides: Lactose-containing foods such as milk, yogurt, and certain soft cheeses fall into this category.

3. Monosaccharides: Foods high in excess fructose, like certain fruits (such as apples, pears, and watermelon) and honey.

4. Polyols: These include sugar alcohols found in some fruits (like cherries, peaches, and blackberries), as well as certain artificial sweeteners (such as sorbitol, mannitol, and xylitol).

Low-FODMAP Foods:

1. Oligosaccharides: Low-FODMAP alternatives include gluten-free grains like rice and quinoa, and green leafy vegetables like spinach and kale.

2. Disaccharides: Lactose-free options like lactose-free milk, hard cheeses (e.g., cheddar, Swiss), and lactose-free yogurts are typically better tolerated.

3. Monosaccharides: Small portions of fruits like strawberries, blueberries, oranges, and grapes are generally considered low in excess fructose.

4. Polyols: Low-FODMAP options include certain fruits like bananas, strawberries, and kiwi, as well as specific sweeteners like glucose and stevia.

The key to successfully following a low-FODMAP diet involves learning which foods fall into each category and tailoring your meals accordingly. It often requires eliminating high-FODMAP foods for a period, followed by systematic reintroduction to pinpoint individual tolerance levels.

Working with a registered dietitian or healthcare professional knowledgeable about the low-FODMAP diet can greatly assist in identifying and navigating high and low FODMAP foods, ensuring a balanced and nutritious diet while minimizing digestive discomfort.

In the realm of the low-FODMAP diet, foods are categorized based on their FODMAP content. High-FODMAP foods, such as certain grains, dairy products, specific fruits, and sweeteners, tend to trigger digestive symptoms in some individuals. On the other hand, low-FODMAP foods, including alternatives like gluten-free grains, lactose-free dairy, select fruits, and specific sweeteners, are better tolerated by many on this diet.

The key to success lies in understanding which foods fall into each category. Learning to identify and differentiate high and low FODMAP foods forms the cornerstone of crafting meals that alleviate digestive discomfort while ensuring proper nutrition and delicious flavors.

Kitchen and Pantry Essentials for a Low-FODMAP Diet

1. Gluten-Free Grains: Stock up on gluten-free alternatives such as rice, quinoa, oats (if tolerated), and cornmeal as versatile staples for meals.

2. Low-FODMAP Flour: Consider having low-FODMAP flours like rice flour, tapioca flour, or potato starch for baking and cooking purposes.

3. Lactose-Free Dairy or Alternatives: Opt for lactose-free milk, hard cheeses (cheddar, Swiss), lactose-free yogurt, or nondairy alternatives like almond milk, coconut yogurt, or lactose-free versions of your preferred dairy products.

4. Low-FODMAP Fruits and Vegetables: Keep a variety of low-FODMAP fruits (bananas, berries, oranges) and vegetables (spinach, kale, bell peppers, carrots) on hand for balanced meals.

5. Protein Sources: Stock up on low-FODMAP protein options such as eggs, tofu, poultry, fish, and canned legumes like chickpeas (drained and rinsed well) in limited amounts.

6. Herbs and Spices: Use fresh or dried herbs and spices like basil, oregano, thyme, turmeric, and cumin to add flavor without FODMAPs.

7. Garlic and Onion Substitutes: Garlic-infused oil or green parts of spring onions (green onions) can be used as flavorful substitutes for garlic and onion in cooking.

8. Low-FODMAP Condiments: Check labels for suitable condiments like mustard, mayonnaise, ketchup, and low-FODMAP sauces or marinades to enhance flavors.

9. Nuts and Seeds: Include low-FODMAP nuts (like almonds and macadamia nuts) and seeds (such as chia seeds or pumpkin seeds) for added nutrition and texture.

10. Low-FODMAP Sweeteners: Choose sweeteners like maple syrup, golden syrup, sugar, or stevia for sweetening, avoiding high-FODMAP options like honey or agave syrup.

11. Gluten-Free Pasta and Bread: Have gluten-free pasta and bread made from rice, corn, or other low-FODMAP grains for meal variety.

12. Canned and Frozen Low-FODMAP Foods: Keep canned tomatoes, canned fish (like tuna or salmon), and frozen low-FODMAP fruits and vegetables as convenient options.

Ensuring a well-stocked kitchen and pantry with these essentials forms the foundation for creating delicious and digestive-friendly meals while adhering to a low-FODMAP diet.

Tips for Grocery Shopping and Meal Planning

1. Plan before Shopping: Outline a meal plan for the week, including breakfast, lunch, dinner, and snacks. This helps in creating a shopping list focused on low-FODMAP ingredients.

2. Read Labels: Carefully read food labels to identify high-FODMAP ingredients and choose suitable alternatives. Look out for hidden sources of FODMAPs like fructose, inulin, or sugar alcohols.

3. Shop the Perimeter: Focus on fresh produce, meats, and dairy or lactose-free alternatives found around the store's perimeter. This typically contains more whole foods and fewer processed items.

4. Choose Low-FODMAP Foods: Prioritize low-FODMAP options such as gluten-free grains (rice, quinoa), low-FODMAP fruits and vegetables (bananas, spinach), lactose-free dairy, and suitable proteins (chicken, fish).

5. Stock up on Pantry Staples: Keep essential pantry items like gluten-free flours, low-FODMAP condiments, herbs, spices, and canned or frozen low-FODMAP foods for convenience.

6. Experiment with Recipes: Explore and experiment with low-FODMAP recipes to add variety to meals. Look for reliable sources such as low-FODMAP cookbooks or reputable websites.

7. Prepare in Advance: Prepping ingredients in advance can save time during the week. Wash, chop, and portion out fruits, vegetables, and proteins for easier meal preparation.

8. Use a Shopping App or List: Utilize apps or create a physical shopping list based on your meal plan and required ingredients to ensure you don't forget anything essential while shopping.

9. Be Mindful of Portions: Some low-FODMAP foods might become high in FODMAPs in larger portions. Be aware of serving sizes and FODMAP content, especially with certain fruits, vegetables, and grains.

10. Allow for Flexibility: Embrace flexibility in meal planning and be open to trying new low-FODMAP ingredients or recipes to keep meals interesting and enjoyable.

By incorporating these tips into your grocery shopping routine and meal planning process, you can streamline the process of finding suitable ingredients and crafting delicious, digestive friendly meals while following a low-FODMAP diet.

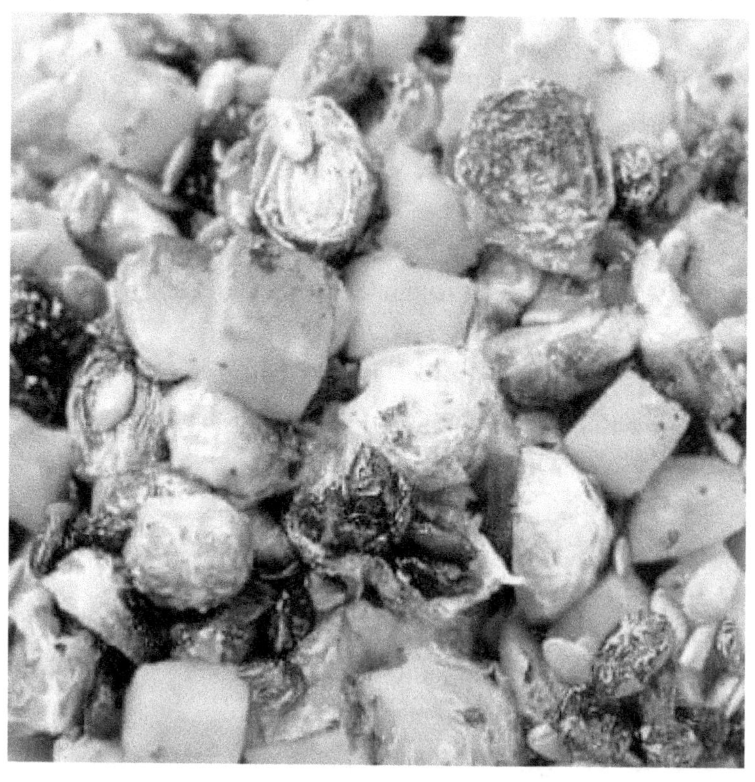

CHAPTER 3

Low-FODMAP Recipes for Digestive Health

DELICIOUS AND NUTRITIOUS MORNING RECIPES

Banana Berry Smoothie

Ingredients:
1 ripe banana
1 cup mixed berries (strawberries, blueberries)
1 cup lactose-free yogurt or almond milk
Ice cubes (optional)

Preparation:
1. Peel and slice the banana.
2. Wash the berries thoroughly.
3. In a blender, combine the banana slices, mixed berries, and lactose-free yogurt or almond milk.
4. Add ice cubes if desired.
Blend until smooth and creamy

Nutritional Value (Approximate):
Calories: 180
Carbohydrates: 40g
Protein: 5g
Fat: 2g

Preparation: 5 minutes

Scrambled Eggs with Spinach

Ingredients:
3 large eggs
1 cup fresh spinach leaves
1 tablespoon lactose-free milk or water
Salt and pepper to taste
Cooking oil (optional)

Preparation:
1. Whisk the eggs and lactose-free milk or water in a bowl.
2. Heat a nonstick skillet over medium heat.
3. Add spinach leaves to the skillet and cook until wilted.
4. Pour the whisked eggs into the skillet.
5. Gently scramble the eggs and spinach until cooked to desired consistency.
6. Season with salt and pepper.

Nutritional Value (Approximate):
Calories: 220
Carbohydrates: 2g
Protein: 18g
Fat: 15g

Preparation and Cooking: 10 minutes

Quinoa Breakfast Bowl

Ingredients:
1/2 cup cooked quinoa
1/4 cup sliced strawberries
1/4 cup blueberries
2 tablespoons chopped almonds or walnuts
1 tablespoon maple syrup

Preparation:
1. Cook quinoa according to package instructions and let it cool.
2. In a bowl, combine cooked quinoa, sliced strawberries, blueberries, and chopped nuts.
3. Drizzle with maple syrup for sweetness.

Nutritional Value (Approximate):
Calories: 280
Carbohydrates: 35g

Protein: 8g
Fat: 12g

Preparation: 10 minutes (if quinoa is precooked)

Low-FODMAP Overnight Oats

Ingredients:
1/2 cup gluten-free oats
1 cup lactose-free milk or almond milk
1 tablespoon chia seeds
1 tablespoon maple syrup
1/4 cup sliced kiwi (optional)

Preparation:
1. In a jar or bowl, combine oats, lactose-free milk, chia seeds, and maple syrup.
2. Stir well, cover, and refrigerate overnight.
3. In the morning, top with sliced kiwi or other tolerated fruits if desired.

Nutritional Value (Approximate):
Calories: 300
Carbohydrates: 45g
Protein: 8g
Fat: 10g

Preparation (plus overnight refrigeration): 5 minutes

Tofu and Vegetable Stir-Fry

Ingredients:
150g firm tofu, cubed
1 cup mixed bell peppers, sliced
1 cup spinach
1 tablespoon low-FODMAP stir-fry sauce
Cooking oil (optional)

Preparation:
1. Heat a nonstick skillet or wok over medium-high heat.
2. Add tofu cubes and cook until lightly browned on all sides.
3. Add sliced bell peppers and stir-fry for 23 minutes.
4. Add spinach and stir-fry until wilted.
5. Pour low-FODMAP stir-fry sauce over the mixture and toss to coat.

Nutritional Value (Approximate):
Calories: 250
Carbohydrates: 12g
Protein: 20g
Fat: 12g

Preparation and Cooking: 15 minutes

Chia Seed Pudding

Ingredients:
2 tablespoons chia seeds
1 cup lactose-free milk or almond milk
1/2 teaspoon vanilla extract
1 tablespoon maple syrup (optional)
Low-FODMAP fruits for topping (e.g., strawberries, kiwi)

Preparation:
1. In a bowl or jar, mix chia seeds, lactose-free milk, vanilla extract, and maple syrup (if using).
2. Stir well and refrigerate for at least 4 hours or overnight until it thickens into a pudding-like consistency.
3. Top with low-FODMAP fruits before serving.

Nutritional Value (Approximate):
Calories: 180
Carbohydrates: 20g
Protein: 5g
Fat: 9g

Preparation (plus chilling time): 5 minutes

Rice Cake with Peanut Butter and Banana

Ingredients:
1 rice cake (gluten-free)
1 tablespoon natural peanut butter
1/2 ripe banana, sliced
Cinnamon powder (optional)

Preparation:
1. Spread peanut butter evenly on the rice cake.
2. Arrange banana slices on top.
3. Sprinkle with a dash of cinnamon if desired.

Nutritional Value (Approximate):
Calories: 180
Carbohydrates: 25g
Protein: 4g
Fat: 7g

Preparation: 3 minutes

Lactose-Free Yogurt Parfait

Ingredients:
1 cup lactose-free yogurt (plain or flavored)
1/4 cup low-FODMAP granola
1/4 cup mixed low-FODMAP berries (e.g., blueberries, raspberries)
1 tablespoon sliced almonds

Preparation:
1. In a glass or bowl, layer lactose-free yogurt, low-FODMAP granola, mixed berries, and sliced almonds.
2. Repeat layers if desired.

Nutritional Value (Approximate):
Calories: 250
Carbohydrates: 30g
Protein: 10g
Fat: 10g

Preparation: 5 minutes

Spinach and Tomato Frittata

Ingredients:
4 large eggs
1 cup fresh spinach leaves
1/2 cup diced tomatoes (fresh or canned, drained)
Salt and pepper to taste
Cooking oil (optional)

Preparation:
1. Preheat oven to 350°F (175°C).
2. In a bowl, whisk eggs and season with salt and pepper.
3. Heat an ovenproof skillet over medium heat, add oil if using.
4. Add spinach and cook until wilted, then add diced tomatoes.
5. Pour the whisked eggs over the vegetables.
6. Cook on the stovetop for a few minutes, then transfer the skillet to the oven and bake until the frittata is set (about 1015 minutes).

Nutritional Value (Approximate):
Calories: 220
Carbohydrates: 4g
Protein: 18g
Fat: 15g

Preparation and Cooking: 20 minutes

Low-FODMAP Breakfast Burrito

Ingredients:
2 gluten-free tortillas
2 large eggs, scrambled
1/4 cup diced bell peppers
2 tablespoons diced green onions (green parts only)
2 tablespoons shredded cheddar cheese (optional)
Cooking oil (optional)

Preparation:
1. Heat a nonstick skillet over medium heat, add oil if desired.
2. Add diced bell peppers and green onions, sauté until softened.
3. Add scrambled eggs and cook until done.
4. Warm tortillas in the skillet or microwave.
5. Divide the egg mixture between the tortillas, add cheese if using, and roll into burritos.

Nutritional Value (Approximate):
Calories: 300
Carbohydrates: 25g
Protein: 15g
Fat: 15g

Preparation and Cooking: 10 minutes

Greek Yogurt Pancakes

Ingredients:
1 cup gluten-free oat flour
1 teaspoon baking powder
1/2 teaspoon cinnamon (optional)
1 cup lactose-free Greek yogurt
2 large eggs
Cooking oil or butter for the skillet

Preparation:
1. In a bowl, whisk together oat flour, baking powder, and cinnamon.
2. In another bowl, mix Greek yogurt and eggs until smooth.
3. Combine the wet and dry ingredients until just mixed.
4. Heat a skillet over medium heat, lightly grease with oil or butter.
5. Pour small amounts of batter onto the skillet to make pancakes.
6. Cook until bubbles form on the surface, then flip and cook the other side.

Nutritional Value (Approximate):
Calories: 250
Carbohydrates: 25g
Protein: 15g
Fat: 10g

Preparation and Cooking: 15 minutes

Tofu Scramble Wrap

Ingredients:
150g firm tofu, crumbled
1/4 cup diced bell peppers
1/4 cup spinach
1 tablespoon low-FODMAP salsa
2 gluten-free tortillas

Preparation:
1. Heat a skillet over medium heat.
2. Add crumbled tofu, bell peppers, and spinach to the skillet.
3. Cook until vegetables are tender and tofu is heated through.
4. Stir in low-FODMAP salsa and cook for another minute.
5. Warm tortillas in a separate skillet or microwave.
6. Divide the tofu scramble between the tortillas, fold, and serve.

Nutritional Value (Approximate):
Calories: 280
Carbohydrates: 30g
Protein: 15g

Fat: 12g

Preparation and Cooking: 10 minutes

Low-FODMAP Breakfast Hash

Ingredients:
2 cups diced potatoes (white or sweet potatoes)
1/2 cup diced bell peppers
1/4 cup diced tomatoes (fresh or canned, drained)
2 tablespoons chopped green onions (green parts only)
Salt, pepper, and paprika to taste
Cooking oil

Preparation:
1. Heat oil in a skillet over medium-high heat.
2. Add diced potatoes and cook until golden and tender.
3. Add bell peppers and continue cooking until slightly softened.
4. Stir in diced tomatoes and green onions, cook for a few more minutes.
5. Season with salt, pepper, and paprika.

Nutritional Value (Approximate):
Calories: 240
Carbohydrates: 35g
Protein: 4g

Fat: 10g

Preparation and Cooking: 20 minutes

Low-FODMAP Avocado Toast

Ingredients:
2 slices gluten-free bread (toasted)
1 ripe avocado
Lemon juice (optional)
Red pepper flakes (optional)
Salt and pepper to taste

Preparation:
1. Toast gluten-free bread slices until golden.
2. Mash the ripe avocado and spread it evenly on the toast.
3. Sprinkle with lemon juice, red pepper flakes, salt, and pepper if desired.

Nutritional Value (Approximate):
Calories: 200
Carbohydrates: 20g
Protein: 4g
Fat: 12g

Preparation: 5 minutes

Low-FODMAP Breakfast Sushi Rolls

Ingredients:
2 nori seaweed sheets
1/2 cup cooked quinoa
1/4 cup sliced cucumber
1/4 cup sliced carrots
2 tablespoons sliced green onions (green parts only)
Low-FODMAP dipping sauce (e.g., soy sauce alternative)

Preparation:
1. Place a nori sheet on a flat surface.
2. Spread cooked quinoa evenly on the nori sheet.
3. Arrange sliced cucumber, carrots, and green onions along one edge.
4. Roll the nori sheet tightly, then slice into sushi rolls.
5. Serve with low-FODMAP dipping sauce.

Nutritional Value (Approximate):
Calories: 180
Carbohydrates: 30g
Protein: 6g
Fat: 4g

Preparation: 15 minutes

NOURISHING AND SATISFYING LUNCH OPTIONS

Grilled Chicken Salad

Ingredients:
2 boneless, skinless chicken breasts
4 cups mixed salad greens (e.g., spinach, lettuce)
1 cup cherry tomatoes, halved
1 cucumber, sliced
1/4 cup sliced carrots
2 tablespoons olive oil
1 tablespoon balsamic vinegar
Salt and pepper to taste

Preparation:
1. Preheat grill or grill pan over medium-high heat.
2. Season chicken breasts with salt and pepper.
3. Grill chicken for about 68 minutes per side until fully cooked.
4. In a bowl, toss salad greens, cherry tomatoes, cucumber, and carrots.
5. Slice grilled chicken and place on top of the salad.

6. Drizzle olive oil and balsamic vinegar over the salad.

Nutritional Value (Approximate):
Calories: 350
Carbohydrates: 10g
Protein: 35g
Fat: 18g

Preparation and Cooking: 20 minutes

Low-FODMAP Turkey Wrap

Ingredients:
2 gluten-free tortillas
6 slices low-FODMAP deli turkey
1 cup mixed salad greens
1/4 cup sliced bell peppers
2 tablespoons lactose-free cream cheese
Salt and pepper to taste

Preparation:
1. Lay out the tortillas and spread lactose-free cream cheese evenly on each.
2. Place three slices of turkey on each tortilla.
3. Top with mixed salad greens and sliced bell peppers.
4. Season with salt and pepper.
5. Roll up the tortillas tightly to form wraps.

Nutritional Value (Approximate):
Calories: 300
Carbohydrates: 25g
Protein: 15g
Fat: 15g

Preparation: 10 minutes

Quinoa and Vegetable Stir-Fry

Ingredients:
1 cup cooked quinoa
1 cup mixed bell peppers, sliced
1 cup zucchini, sliced
1 cup spinach leaves
2 tablespoons low-FODMAP stir-fry sauce
2 tablespoons olive oil
Salt and pepper to taste

Preparation:
1. Heat olive oil in a skillet over medium-high heat.
2. Add mixed bell peppers and zucchini, stir-fry for 34 minutes.
3. Add spinach leaves and cooked quinoa to the skillet.
4. Pour low-FODMAP stir-fry sauce over the mixture.
5. Stir-fry until everything is heated through.

6. Season with salt and pepper.

Nutritional Value (Approximate):
Calories: 320
Carbohydrates: 35g
Protein: 8g
Fat: 16g

Preparation and Cooking: 15 minutes

Low-FODMAP Tuna Salad

Ingredients:
2 cans (5 oz. each) canned tuna in water, drained
1/4 cup diced red bell pepper
1/4 cup diced cucumber
2 tablespoons chopped green onions (green parts only)
2 tablespoons mayonnaise (check for low-FODMAP ingredients)
1 tablespoon lemon juice
Salt and pepper to taste

Preparation:
1. In a bowl, combine drained tuna, diced bell pepper, cucumber, and green onions.
2. Add mayonnaise and lemon juice, mix well.

3. Season with salt and pepper to taste.

4. Serve on a bed of lettuce or as a sandwich filling.

Nutritional Value (Approximate):
Calories: 250
Carbohydrates: 4g
Protein: 30g
Fat: 12g

Preparation: 10 minutes

Baked Salmon with Roasted Vegetables

Ingredients:
2 salmon fillets (6 oz. each)
2 cups mixed low-FODMAP vegetables (e.g., bell peppers, zucchini, and carrots)
2 tablespoons olive oil
Salt, pepper, and herbs (such as thyme or rosemary) to taste
Lemon wedges for serving

Preparation:
1. Preheat oven to 400°F (200°C).

2. Place salmon fillets on a baking sheet lined with parchment paper.

3. Toss mixed vegetables with olive oil, salt, pepper, and herbs.

4. Spread vegetables around the salmon on the baking sheet.

5. Bake in the preheated oven for 1520 minutes until salmon is cooked through and vegetables are tender.

6. Serve with lemon wedges.

Nutritional Value (Approximate):
Calories: 380
Carbohydrates: 10g
Protein: 35g
Fat: 22g

Preparation and Cooking: 25 minutes

Quinoa Salad with Lemon-Herb Dressing

Ingredients:
1 cup cooked quinoa
1 cup diced cucumbers
1 cup cherry tomatoes, halved
1/4 cup chopped fresh parsley
2 tablespoons chopped fresh mint
2 tablespoons olive oil
1 tablespoon lemon juice

Salt and pepper to taste

Preparation:
1. In a bowl, combine cooked quinoa, diced cucumbers, cherry tomatoes, parsley, and mint.
2. In a small bowl, whisk together olive oil, lemon juice, salt, and pepper to make the dressing.
3. Pour the dressing over the quinoa salad and toss gently to combine.
4. Serve chilled.

Nutritional Value (Approximate):
Calories: 280
Carbohydrates: 30g
Protein: 5g
Fat: 15g

Preparation: 15 minutes

Low-FODMAP Turkey and Veggie Skewers

Ingredients:
8 oz. low-FODMAP deli turkey, cut into cubes
1 cup bell peppers (assorted colors), cut into chunks
1 cup zucchini, sliced

1 cup cherry tomatoes
2 tablespoons olive oil
1 tablespoon low-FODMAP Italian seasoning
Salt and pepper to taste

Preparation:
1. Preheat grill or grill pan over medium-high heat.
2. Thread the turkey cubes, bell peppers, zucchini, and cherry tomatoes onto skewers.
3. In a bowl, mix olive oil, Italian seasoning, salt, and pepper.
4. Brush the skewers with the olive oil mixture.
5. Grill the skewers for about 810 minutes, turning occasionally, until turkey is cooked and vegetables are tender.
6. Serve hot.

Nutritional Value (Approximate):
Calories: 280
Carbohydrates: 10g
Protein: 25g
Fat: 15g

Preparation and Cooking: 15 minutes

Eggplant and Tomato Pasta

Ingredients:

8 oz. gluten-free pasta

1 medium eggplant, diced

1 cup cherry tomatoes, halved

2 tablespoons olive oil

2 cloves garlic, minced

1/4 cup fresh basil leaves, chopped

Salt and pepper to taste

Preparation:

1. Cook gluten-free pasta according to package instructions.

2. Heat olive oil in a skillet over medium heat.

3. Add diced eggplant and cook until softened.

4. Add cherry tomatoes and minced garlic, cook for 34 minutes.

5. Season with salt and pepper.

6. Toss cooked pasta with the eggplant, tomato mixture.

7. Sprinkle chopped basil on top before serving.

Nutritional Value (Approximate):

Calories: 320

Carbohydrates: 45g

Protein: 6g

Fat: 14g

Preparation and Cooking: 25 minutes

Low-FODMAP Chicken Lettuce Wraps

Ingredients:
1 lb. ground chicken
1 cup shredded carrots
1 cup chopped water chestnuts
2 tablespoons low-FODMAP stir-fry sauce
2 tablespoons green onions (green parts only), chopped
Iceberg lettuce leaves for wrapping

Preparation:
1. Heat a skillet over medium-high heat.
2. Add ground chicken and cook until browned.
3. Stir in shredded carrots, water chestnuts, and stir-fry sauce.
4. Cook for 34 minutes until heated through.
5. Sprinkle chopped green onions on top.
6. Spoon the chicken mixture into lettuce leaves and serve.

Nutritional Value (Approximate):
Calories: 290
Carbohydrates: 10g
Protein: 25g

Fat: 15g

Preparation and Cooking: 20 minutes

Lentil and Vegetable Soup

Ingredients:
1 cup lentils (rinsed)
4 cups low-FODMAP vegetable broth
1 cup diced carrots
1 cup diced potatoes
1 cup diced zucchini
2 tablespoons olive oil
2 cloves garlic, minced
1 teaspoon dried thyme
Salt and pepper to taste

Preparation:
1. In a large pot, heat olive oil over medium heat.
2. Add minced garlic and cook until fragrant.
3. Add diced carrots, potatoes, and zucchini. Cook for 5 minutes.
4. Stir in lentils, vegetable broth, dried thyme, salt, and pepper.
5. Bring to a boil, then reduce heat and simmer for 2025 minutes until lentils and vegetables are tender.
6. Serve hot.

Nutritional Value (Approximate):
Calories: 280
Carbohydrates: 45g
Protein: 15g
Fat: 7g

Preparation and Cooking: 35 minutes

Low-FODMAP Chicken and Vegetable Stir-Fry

Ingredients:
2 boneless, skinless chicken breasts, sliced
1 cup bell peppers (assorted colors), sliced
1 cup carrots, sliced
1 cup bok choy, chopped
2 tablespoons low-FODMAP stir-fry sauce
2 tablespoons olive oil
Salt and pepper to taste

Preparation:
1. Heat olive oil in a skillet or wok over medium-high heat.
2. Add sliced chicken breasts and cook until browned.
3. Stir in sliced bell peppers, carrots, and bok choy.
4. Cook for 45 minutes until vegetables are tender crisp.

5. Add low-FODMAP stir-fry sauce, and toss to coat evenly.
6. Season with salt and pepper.
7. Serve hot.

Nutritional Value (Approximate):
Calories: 320
Carbohydrates: 12g
Protein: 30g
Fat: 15g

Preparation and Cooking: 20 minutes

Low-FODMAP Veggie Quesadilla

Ingredients:
2 gluten-free tortillas
1 cup shredded cheddar cheese
1 cup sliced bell peppers (assorted colors)
1 cup spinach leaves
Cooking oil for the skillet

Preparation:
1. Heat a skillet over medium heat, add a tortilla.
2. Sprinkle half of the shredded cheese over the tortilla.
3. Layer sliced bell peppers and spinach on top of the cheese.
4. Sprinkle the remaining cheese over the vegetables.
5. Place the second tortilla on top.

6. Cook until the bottom tortilla is golden and cheese melts.

7. Flip and cook the other side until golden.

8. Remove from heat, slice into wedges, and serve.

Nutritional Value (Approximate):
Calories: 350
Carbohydrates: 25g
Protein: 15g
Fat: 20g

Preparation and Cooking: 15 minutes

Low-FODMAP Tofu Lettuce Wraps

Ingredients:
1 block firm tofu, crumbled
1 cup shredded carrots
1 cup chopped water chestnuts
2 tablespoons low-FODMAP soy sauce
2 tablespoons green onions (green parts only), chopped
Iceberg lettuce leaves for wrapping

Preparation:
1. Heat a skillet over medium-high heat.
2. Add crumbled tofu and cook until slightly browned.
3. Stir in shredded carrots, water chestnuts, and soy sauce.
4. Cook for 34 minutes until heated through.

5. Sprinkle chopped green onions on top.
6. Spoon the tofu mixture into lettuce leaves and serve.

Nutritional Value (Approximate):
Calories: 260
Carbohydrates: 20g
Protein: 15g
Fat: 12g

Preparation and Cooking: 20 minutes

Low-FODMAP Egg Fried Rice

Ingredients:
2 cups cooked white rice (cooled)
2 eggs, beaten
1 cup mixed vegetables (e.g., peas, carrots)
2 tablespoons low-FODMAP soy sauce
2 tablespoons chopped green onions (green parts only)
2 tablespoons olive oil
Salt and pepper to taste

Preparation:
1. Heat olive oil in a skillet over medium heat.
2. Add beaten eggs and scramble until cooked.
3. Stir in mixed vegetables and cooked rice.

4. Add low-FODMAP soy sauce, green onions, salt, and pepper.
5. Cook and stir for 34 minutes until heated through.
6. Serve hot.

Nutritional Value (Approximate):
Calories: 300
Carbohydrates: 40g
Protein: 8g
Fat: 12g

Preparation and Cooking: 15 minutes

Low-FODMAP Greek-Style Quinoa Bowl

Ingredients:
1 cup cooked quinoa
1 cup cherry tomatoes, halved
1 cucumber, diced
1/2 cup pitted kalamata olives, sliced
1/4 cup crumbled feta cheese (optional)
2 tablespoons olive oil
1 tablespoon red wine vinegar
Fresh oregano (or dried) for garnish
Salt and pepper to taste

Preparation:

1. In a bowl, combine cooked quinoa, cherry tomatoes, diced cucumber, and sliced olives.
2. Drizzle olive oil and red wine vinegar over the mixture.
3. Add crumbled feta cheese if using.
4. Season with salt, pepper, and garnish with fresh oregano.
5. Toss gently to combine.
6. Serve at room temperature.

Nutritional Value (Approximate):
Calories: 280
Carbohydrates: 30g
Protein: 6g
Fat: 15g

Preparation: 10 minutes

FLAVORFUL AND EASY-TO-PREPARE DINNER RECIPES

Grilled Lemon Herb Chicken

Ingredients:
4 boneless, skinless chicken breasts
2 tablespoons olive oil
2 tablespoons fresh lemon juice
2 cloves garlic, minced
1 tablespoon chopped fresh parsley
1 teaspoon dried thyme
Salt and pepper to taste

Preparation:
1. In a bowl, mix olive oil, lemon juice, minced garlic, chopped parsley, dried thyme, salt, and pepper.
2. Marinate chicken breasts in the mixture for 30 minutes.
3. Preheat grill to medium-high heat.
4. Grill chicken for about 68 minutes per side until fully cooked.
5. Serve hot.

Nutritional Value (Approximate):
Calories: 280

Carbohydrates: 1g
Protein: 35g
Fat: 14g

Preparation and Cooking: 20 minutes

Low-FODMAP Baked Salmon with Herbs

Ingredients:
4 salmon fillets (6 oz. each)
2 tablespoons olive oil
2 tablespoons chopped fresh dill
2 tablespoons chopped fresh parsley
1 tablespoon fresh lemon juice
Salt and pepper to taste

Preparation:
1. Preheat oven to 400°F (200°C).
2. Place salmon fillets on a baking sheet lined with parchment paper.
3. Mix olive oil, chopped dill, chopped parsley, lemon juice, salt, and pepper in a bowl.
4. Brush the herb mixture over the salmon fillets.
5. Bake in the preheated oven for 1215 minutes until salmon is cooked through.

6. Serve hot.

Nutritional Value (Approximate):
Calories: 320
Carbohydrates: 0g
Protein: 35g
Fat: 20g

Preparation and Cooking: 20 minutes

Low-FODMAP Turkey Meatballs with Tomato Sauce

Ingredients:
1 lb. ground turkey
1/4 cup gluten-free breadcrumbs
1 egg
1/4 cup chopped fresh parsley
1/4 cup chopped green onions (green parts only)
2 cups low-FODMAP tomato sauce
2 tablespoons olive oil
Salt and pepper to taste

Preparation:
1. Preheat oven to 375°F (190°C).

2. In a bowl, mix ground turkey, gluten-free breadcrumbs, egg, chopped parsley, chopped green onions, salt, and pepper.

3. Shape the mixture into meatballs and place on a baking sheet.

4. Bake meatballs in the preheated oven for 2025 minutes until cooked through.

5. Heat olive oil in a skillet over medium heat, add tomato sauce and bring to a simmer.

6. Add cooked meatballs to the sauce and simmer for an additional 5 minutes.

7. Serve hot.

Nutritional Value (Approximate):
Calories: 280
Carbohydrates: 10g
Protein: 30g
Fat: 15g

Preparation and Cooking: 35 minutes

Low-FODMAP Stir-Fried Shrimp and Vegetables

Ingredients:
1 lb. shrimp, peeled and deveined
2 cups mixed vegetables (bell peppers, broccoli, and carrots)
2 tablespoons low-FODMAP stir-fry sauce
2 tablespoons olive oil
2 cloves garlic, minced
Salt and pepper to taste

Preparation:
1. Heat olive oil in a wok or skillet over high heat.
2. Add minced garlic and stir-fry for 30 seconds.
3. Add shrimp and cook until they turn pink and opaque.
4. Add mixed vegetables and stir-fry for 34 minutes until tender-crisp.
5. Pour low-FODMAP stir-fry sauce over the mixture.
6. Stir-fry for an additional minute.
7. Season with salt and pepper.
8. Serve hot.

Nutritional Value (Approximate):
Calories: 260
Carbohydrates: 10g
Protein: 25g

Fat: 12g

Preparation and Cooking: 15 minutes

Low-FODMAP Quinoa Stuffed Bell Peppers

Ingredients:
4 bell peppers, halved and seeds removed
1 cup cooked quinoa
1 cup diced tomatoes (canned, drained)
1 cup chopped spinach
1/4 cup chopped fresh basil
1/4 cup shredded cheddar cheese (optional)
2 tablespoons olive oil
Salt and pepper to taste

Preparation:
1. Preheat oven to 375°F (190°C).
2. In a bowl, mix cooked quinoa, diced tomatoes, chopped spinach, chopped basil, salt, and pepper.
3. Drizzle olive oil over the bell pepper halves and place them on a baking dish.
4. Fill each bell pepper half with the quinoa mixture.
5. If using, sprinkle shredded cheddar cheese on top of each stuffed pepper.

6. Cover the baking dish with foil and bake in the preheated oven for 2530 minutes until the peppers are tender.

7. Remove the foil and bake for an additional 510 minutes until the cheese (if added) is melted and slightly golden.

8. Serve hot.

Nutritional Value (Approximate):
Calories: 240
Carbohydrates: 30g
Protein: 7g
Fat: 10g

Preparation and Cooking: 40-45 minutes

Low-FODMAP Beef and Vegetable Stir-Fry

Ingredients:
1 lb. beef sirloin, thinly sliced
2 cups mixed vegetables (snap peas, bell peppers, carrots)
2 tablespoons low-FODMAP stir-fry sauce
2 tablespoons olive oil
2 cloves garlic, minced
Salt and pepper to taste

Preparation:

1. Heat olive oil in a wok or skillet over high heat.
2. Add minced garlic and stir-fry for 30 seconds.
3. Add sliced beef and cook until browned.
4. Add mixed vegetables and stir-fry for 34 minutes until tender-crisp.
5. Pour low-FODMAP stir-fry sauce over the mixture.
6. Stir-fry for an additional minute.
7. Season with salt and pepper.
8. Serve hot.

Nutritional Value (Approximate):
Calories: 320
Carbohydrates: 8g
Protein: 30g
Fat: 18g

Preparation and Cooking: 20 minutes

Low-FODMAP Pesto Chicken Pasta

Ingredients:
8 oz. gluten-free pasta
2 boneless, skinless chicken breasts, diced
1/4 cup low-FODMAP pesto sauce
1 cup cherry tomatoes, halved
2 tablespoons olive oil

Salt and pepper to taste

Preparation:
1. Cook gluten-free pasta according to package instructions.
2. Heat olive oil in a skillet over medium-high heat.
3. Add diced chicken breasts and cook until browned.
4. Reduce heat, add cherry tomatoes, and cook for 34 minutes.
5. Stir in low-FODMAP pesto sauce.
6. Add cooked pasta to the skillet and toss to coat.
7. Season with salt and pepper.
8. Serve hot.

Nutritional Value (Approximate):
Calories: 380
Carbohydrates: 40g
Protein: 25g
Fat: 15g

Preparation and Cooking: 25 minutes

Low-FODMAP Veggie Pizza

Ingredients:
1 gluten-free pizza crust
1/2 cup low-FODMAP pizza sauce
1 cup shredded mozzarella cheese

1 cup mixed vegetables (bell peppers, tomatoes, olives)
2 tablespoons olive oil
Fresh basil leaves for garnish
Salt and pepper to taste

Preparation:
1. Preheat oven according to pizza crust instructions.
2. Spread low-FODMAP pizza sauce evenly on the crust.
3. Sprinkle shredded mozzarella cheese over the sauce.
4. Top with mixed vegetables.
5. Drizzle olive oil over the vegetables.
6. Season with salt and pepper.
7. Bake in the preheated oven as per the crust instructions until the cheese is melted and bubbly.
8. Garnish with fresh basil leaves.
9. Slice and serve.

Nutritional Value (Approximate):
Calories: 300
Carbohydrates: 35g
Protein: 10g
Fat: 15g

Preparation and Cooking: Varies based on pizza crust

Low-FODMAP Stuffed Zucchini Boats

Ingredients:
4 medium zucchinis
1 cup cooked quinoa
1 cup diced bell peppers
1 cup chopped spinach
1/4 cup shredded cheddar cheese (optional)
2 tablespoons olive oil
Salt and pepper to taste

Preparation:
1. Preheat oven to 375°F (190°C).
2. Cut zucchinis in half lengthwise and scoop out the flesh to form boats.
3. In a bowl, mix cooked quinoa, diced bell peppers, chopped spinach, salt, and pepper.
4. Fill each zucchini boat with the quinoa mixture.
5. If using, sprinkle shredded cheddar cheese on top of each boat.
6. Place the boats on a baking dish, drizzle olive oil over them.
7. Bake in the preheated oven for 2025 minutes until zucchinis are tender.
8. Serve hot.

Nutritional Value (Approximate):
Calories: 220
Carbohydrates: 25g
Protein: 8g
Fat: 12g

Preparation and Cooking: 30 minutes

Low-FODMAP Asian-Inspired Tofu Stir-Fry

Ingredients:
1 block firm tofu, cut into cubes
2 cups mixed vegetables (broccoli, bell peppers, snow peas)
2 tablespoons low-FODMAP stir-fry sauce
2 tablespoons sesame oil
2 cloves garlic, minced
Salt and pepper to taste

Preparation:
1. Heat sesame oil in a skillet or wok over medium-high heat.
2. Add minced garlic and stir-fry for 30 seconds.
3. Add tofu cubes and cook until lightly browned.
4. Add mixed vegetables and stir-fry for 45 minutes until tender-crisp.
5. Pour low-FODMAP stir-fry sauce over the mixture.

6. Stir-fry for an additional minute.
7. Season with salt and pepper.
8. Serve hot.

Nutritional Value (Approximate):
Calories: 280
Carbohydrates: 15g
Protein: 15g
Fat: 18g

Preparation and Cooking: 20 minutes

Low-FODMAP Turkey Chili

Ingredients:
1 lb. ground turkey
1 can (15 oz.) diced tomatoes (low-FODMAP)
1 can (15 oz.) red kidney beans, drained and rinsed
1 cup diced bell peppers
1 cup chopped carrots
1 cup low-FODMAP vegetable broth
2 tablespoons olive oil
2 cloves garlic, minced
2 teaspoons cumin
1 teaspoon paprika
Salt and pepper to taste

Preparation:

1. Heat olive oil in a large pot over medium heat.

2. Add minced garlic and sauté for 1 minute.

3. Add ground turkey and cook until browned.

4. Stir in diced tomatoes, kidney beans, bell peppers, carrots, vegetable broth, cumin, paprika, salt, and pepper.

5. Bring to a boil, then reduce heat and simmer for 2530 minutes.

6. Serve hot, optionally garnished with chopped green onions or parsley.

Nutritional Value (Approximate):

Calories: 320

Carbohydrates: 30g

Protein: 25g

Fat: 12g

Preparation and Cooking: 45 minutes

Low-FODMAP Lemon Garlic Shrimp Pasta

Ingredients:

8 oz. gluten-free pasta

1 lb. shrimp, peeled and deveined

2 tablespoons olive oil

2 cloves garlic, minced
Zest of 1 lemon
Juice of 1 lemon
1/4 cup chopped fresh parsley
Salt and pepper to taste

Preparation:
1. Cook gluten-free pasta according to package instructions.
2. Heat olive oil in a skillet over medium heat.
3. Add minced garlic and sauté for 1 minute.
4. Add shrimp and cook until pink and opaque.
5. Stir in lemon zest, lemon juice, chopped parsley, salt, and pepper.
6. Toss cooked pasta with the shrimp mixture.
7. Serve hot.

Nutritional Value (Approximate):
Calories: 330
Carbohydrates: 35g
Protein: 25g
Fat: 12g

Preparation and Cooking: 20 minutes

Low-FODMAP Baked Chicken Thighs

Ingredients:
4 chicken thighs, bone-in, skin-on
2 tablespoons olive oil
2 teaspoons paprika
1 teaspoon dried thyme
1 teaspoon garlic powder
Salt and pepper to taste

Preparation:
1. Preheat oven to 400°F (200°C).
2. Pat dry chicken thighs with paper towels.
3. In a bowl, mix olive oil, paprika, dried thyme, garlic powder, salt, and pepper.
4. Rub the spice mixture evenly over the chicken thighs.
5. Place chicken thighs on a baking sheet lined with parchment paper.
6. Bake in the preheated oven for 3540 minutes until chicken is fully cooked and skin is crispy.
7. Serve hot.

Nutritional Value (Approximate):
Calories: 280
Carbohydrates: 0g
Protein: 25g

Fat: 18g

Preparation and Cooking: 40 minutes

Low-FODMAP Quinoa and Black Bean Stuffed Peppers

Ingredients:
4 bell peppers, tops removed and seeds removed
1 cup cooked quinoa
1 can (15 oz.) black beans, drained and rinsed
1 cup diced tomatoes (low-FODMAP)
1/2 cup diced red onions (green parts only)
1 teaspoon cumin
1 teaspoon smoked paprika
1/4 cup chopped cilantro
Salt and pepper to taste

Preparation:
1. Preheat oven to 375°F (190°C).
2. In a bowl, mix cooked quinoa, black beans, diced tomatoes, diced red onions, cumin, smoked paprika, chopped cilantro, salt, and pepper.
3. Fill each bell pepper with the quinoa mixture.
4. Place stuffed peppers in a baking dish.

5. Cover the dish with foil and bake in the preheated oven for 2530 minutes until peppers are tender.
6. Serve hot.

Nutritional Value (Approximate):
Calories: 270
Carbohydrates: 45g
Protein: 12g
Fat: 3g

Preparation and Cooking: 40 minutes

Low-FODMAP Ratatouille

Ingredients:
1 eggplant, diced
2 zucchinis, diced
2 bell peppers, diced
2 tomatoes, diced
1 onion, diced
2 cloves garlic, minced
2 tablespoons olive oil
1 teaspoon dried basil
1 teaspoon dried thyme
Salt and pepper to taste

Preparation:
1. Heat olive oil in a large pot over medium heat.
2. Add minced garlic and diced onion, sauté for 23 minutes.
3. Add diced eggplant, zucchinis, bell peppers, and tomatoes to the pot.
4. Stir in dried basil, dried thyme, salt, and pepper.
5. Cook covered for 2025 minutes, stirring occasionally until vegetables are tender.
6. Serve hot as a side dish or main course.

Nutritional Value (Approximate):
Calories: 180
Carbohydrates: 25g
Protein: 4g
Fat: 8g

Preparation and Cooking: 30 minutes

SNACKS AND SMALL BITES

Low-FODMAP Greek Yogurt Parfait

Ingredients:
1 cup lactose-free Greek yogurt
1/2 cup fresh strawberries, sliced
1/4 cup blueberries
2 tablespoons chopped almonds
1 tablespoon maple syrup (optional)

Preparation:
1. In a glass or bowl, layer Greek yogurt, sliced strawberries, and blueberries.
2. Top with chopped almonds.
3. Drizzle with maple syrup if desired.
4. Serve immediately.

Nutritional Value (Approximate):
Calories: 200
Carbohydrates: 20g
Protein: 15g
Fat: 8g

Preparation Time: 5 minutes

Low-FODMAP Rice Cake with Peanut Butter and Banana

Ingredients:
1 rice cake
1 tablespoon peanut butter (ensure no added high-FODMAP ingredients)
1/2 ripe banana, sliced

Preparation:
1. Spread peanut butter evenly over the rice cake.
2. Top with sliced banana.
3. Serve immediately.

Nutritional Value (Approximate):
Calories: 150
Carbohydrates: 20g
Protein: 4g
Fat: 7g

Preparation Time: 2 minutes

Low-FODMAP Caprese Skewers

Ingredients:
Cherry tomatoes
Fresh basil leaves
Mozzarella cheese, cut into cubes
Olive oil (for drizzling)
Balsamic glaze (optional)

Preparation:
1. Thread cherry tomatoes, basil leaves, and mozzarella cubes onto skewers.
2. Drizzle with olive oil and balsamic glaze if desired.
3. Serve immediately.

Nutritional Value (Approximate):
Calories: 120
Carbohydrates: 2g
Protein: 8g
Fat: 9g

Preparation Time: 10 minutes

Low-FODMAP Trail Mix

Ingredients:
1/4 cup mixed nuts (almonds, walnuts, pecans)
2 tablespoons pumpkin seeds
2 tablespoons sunflower seeds
2 tablespoons dark chocolate chips (check for no high-FODMAP additives)

Preparation:
1. Mix all ingredients together in a bowl.
2. Portion into snack-sized bags for easy grab-and-go.

Nutritional Value (Approximate):
Calories: 250
Carbohydrates: 10g
Protein: 8g
Fat: 20g

Preparation Time: 3 minutes

Low-FODMAP Veggie Sticks with Hummus

Ingredients:
Carrot sticks
Cucumber sticks
Red bell pepper strips
Low-FODMAP hummus for dipping

Preparation:
1. Cut carrots, cucumbers, and red bell peppers into sticks/strips.
2. Serve with low-FODMAP hummus for dipping.

Nutritional Value (Approximate):
Calories: 100
Carbohydrates: 15g
Protein: 4g
Fat: 5g

Preparation Time: 5 minutes

Low-FODMAP Tuna Lettuce Wraps

Ingredients:
Canned tuna (in water), drained
Green leaf lettuce leaves
1/4 cup diced tomatoes
1/4 cup diced cucumbers
1 tablespoon mayonnaise (ensure no high-FODMAP ingredients)
Salt and pepper to taste

Preparation:
1. In a bowl, mix drained tuna, diced tomatoes, diced cucumbers, mayonnaise, salt, and pepper.
2. Spoon the tuna mixture onto lettuce leaves.
3. Roll the leaves to create wraps.
4. Serve immediately.

Nutritional Value (Approximate):
Calories: 150
Carbohydrates: 5g
Protein: 15g
Fat: 8g

Preparation Time: 10 minutes

Low-FODMAP Baked Sweet Potato Chips

Ingredients:
2 medium sweet potatoes, thinly sliced
2 tablespoons olive oil
Salt and pepper to taste

Preparation:
1. Preheat oven to 375°F (190°C).
2. Toss sweet potato slices with olive oil, salt, and pepper.
3. Place slices on a baking sheet lined with parchment paper.
4. Bake for 2025 minutes until chips are crispy.
5. Allow to cool before serving.

Nutritional Value (Approximate):
Calories: 120
Carbohydrates: 20g
Protein: 2g
Fat: 5g

Preparation Time: 30 minutes

DESSERTS AND TREATS RECIPES

Low-FODMAP Chocolate Banana Smoothie Bowl

Ingredients:
1 ripe banana
1 tablespoon unsweetened cocoa powder
1/2 cup lactose-free Greek yogurt
1/4 cup almond milk (or other low-FODMAP milk)
1 tablespoon chia seeds (optional)
Toppings: Sliced strawberries, shredded coconut, dark chocolate chips (check for no high-FODMAP additives)

Preparation:
1. Blend ripe banana, cocoa powder, Greek yogurt, almond milk, and chia seeds until smooth.
2. Pour the mixture into a bowl.
3. Top with sliced strawberries, shredded coconut, and dark chocolate chips.
4. Serve immediately.

Nutritional Value (Approximate):
Calories: 250
Carbohydrates: 40g
Protein: 10g
Fat: 8g

Preparation Time: 5 minutes

Low-FODMAP Berry Chia Seed Pudding

Ingredients:
1/4 cup chia seeds
1 cup lactose-free milk
1 tablespoon maple syrup (optional)
1/2 cup mixed berries (strawberries, blueberries, raspberries)
2 tablespoons sliced almonds

Preparation:
1. In a bowl, mix chia seeds, lactose-free milk, and maple syrup.
2. Let it sit in the refrigerator for at least 2 hours or overnight to thicken.
3. Layer chia seed pudding with mixed berries in serving glasses.

4. Top with sliced almonds before serving.

Nutritional Value (Approximate):
Calories: 200
Carbohydrates: 20g
Protein: 6g
Fat: 10g

Preparation Time: 5 minutes (+ chilling time)

Low-FODMAP Peanut Butter Banana Oat Cookies

Ingredients:
2 ripe bananas, mashed
1 cup rolled oats
1/4 cup peanut butter (ensure no high-FODMAP additives)
1/4 cup dark chocolate chips (check for no high-FODMAP additives)
1 teaspoon cinnamon
Pinch of salt

Preparation:
1. Preheat oven to 350°F (175°C).
2. In a bowl, mix mashed bananas, rolled oats, peanut butter, dark chocolate chips, cinnamon, and a pinch of salt.

3. Drop spoonful's of the mixture onto a baking sheet lined with parchment paper.
4. Flatten each cookie with a fork.
5. Bake for 1215 minutes until golden.
6. Allow to cool before serving.

Nutritional Value (Approximate) per cookie (makes about 12 cookies):
Calories: 100
Carbohydrates: 15g
Protein: 3g
Fat: 4g

Preparation Time: 20 minutes

Low-FODMAP Coconut Rice Pudding

Ingredients:
1 cup cooked white rice
1 1/2 cups coconut milk (low-FODMAP)
2 tablespoons maple syrup (optional)
1 teaspoon vanilla extract
1/4 cup shredded coconut
Ground cinnamon for garnish

Preparation:

1. In a saucepan, combine cooked white rice, coconut milk, maple syrup, and vanilla extract.

2. Bring to a simmer over medium heat and cook for 1520 minutes, stirring occasionally, until thickened.

3. Stir in shredded coconut.

4. Remove from heat and let it cool.

5. Serve chilled or at room temperature, garnished with ground cinnamon.

Nutritional Value (Approximate):

Calories: 220

Carbohydrates: 25g

Protein: 2g

Fat: 12g

Preparation Time: 25 minutes

Low-FODMAP Mixed Berry Sorbet

Ingredients:

3 cups mixed berries (strawberries, blueberries, raspberries)

1/4 cup maple syrup (adjust to taste)

1 tablespoon fresh lemon juice

Preparation:
1. Blend mixed berries, maple syrup, and fresh lemon juice until smooth.
2. Pour the mixture into a shallow dish.
3. Freeze for 34 hours, stirring every 30 minutes until firm.
4. Serve scoops of sorbet in dessert bowls.

Nutritional Value (Approximate):
Calories: 150
Carbohydrates: 35g
Protein: 2g
Fat: 1g

Preparation Time:
10 minutes (+ freezing time)

Low-FODMAP Banana Almond Butter Bites

Ingredients:
2 ripe bananas, sliced
2 tablespoons almond butter (ensure no high-FODMAP additives)
1/4 cup shredded coconut
1/4 cup chopped almonds

Preparation:

1. Spread almond butter on banana slices.
2. Sandwich them together to form bites.
3. Roll the edges in shredded coconut and chopped almonds.
4. Refrigerate for 30 minutes before serving.

Nutritional Value (Approximate):

Calories: 160

Carbohydrates: 18g

Protein: 4g

Fat: 10g

Preparation Time:

10 minutes (+ chilling time)

Low-FODMAP Lemon Blueberry Muffins

Ingredients:

1 1/2 cups gluten-free flour

1/2 cup almond flour

1/2 cup maple syrup

1/4 cup melted coconut oil

1/2 cup lactose-free milk

2 eggs

Zest of 1 lemon

Juice of 1 lemon
1 teaspoon baking powder
1/2 teaspoon baking soda
1 cup fresh blueberries

Preparation:
1. Preheat oven to 350°F (175°C). Line a muffin tin with paper liners.
2. In a bowl, whisk together gluten-free flour, almond flour, baking powder, and baking soda.
3. In another bowl, mix maple syrup, melted coconut oil, lactose-free milk, eggs, lemon zest, and lemon juice.
4. Combine wet and dry ingredients until just combined.
5. Gently fold in fresh blueberries.
6. Divide the batter evenly among the muffin cups.
7. Bake for 1820 minutes until a toothpick inserted into the center comes out clean.
8. Allow muffins to cool before serving.

Nutritional Value (Approximate) per muffin (makes about 12 muffins):
Calories: 180
Carbohydrates: 22g
Protein: 4g
Fat: 9g

Preparation Time: 30 minutes

BEVERAGES AND DRINKS RECIPES

Low-FODMAP Strawberry Mint Infused Water

Ingredients:
1 cup sliced strawberries
56 fresh mint leaves
6 cups water
Ice cubes

Preparation:
1. In a pitcher, combine sliced strawberries and fresh mint leaves.
2. Fill the pitcher with 6 cups of water.
3. Refrigerate for at least 2 hours to allow flavors to infuse.
4. Serve over ice.

Nutritional Value (Approximate):
Calories: 5
Carbohydrates: 1g
Protein: 0g
Fat: 0g

Preparation Time: 5 minutes (+ infusing time)

Low-FODMAP Iced Green Tea with Lemon

Ingredients:
4 green tea bags
6 cups hot water
2 tablespoons fresh lemon juice
Ice cubes
Fresh lemon slices for garnish

Preparation:
1. Steep green tea bags in hot water for 34 minutes.
2. Remove tea bags and let the tea cool to room temperature.
3. Stir in fresh lemon juice.
4. Refrigerate until chilled.
5. Serve over ice with fresh lemon slices.

Nutritional Value (Approximate):
Calories: 5
Carbohydrates: 1g
Protein: 0g
Fat: 0g

Preparation Time: 10 minutes (+ chilling time)

Low-FODMAP Pineapple Ginger Smoothie

Ingredients:
1 cup fresh pineapple chunks
1/2 cup lactose-free Greek yogurt
1/2 cup coconut water
1 teaspoon grated fresh ginger
Ice cubes

Preparation:
1. Blend fresh pineapple chunks, lactose-free Greek yogurt, coconut water, and grated fresh ginger until smooth.
2. Add ice cubes and blend again until desired consistency.
3. Serve immediately.

Nutritional Value (Approximate):
Calories: 120
Carbohydrates: 20g
Protein: 8g
Fat: 1g

Preparation Time: 5 minutes

Low-FODMAP Raspberry Lime Sparkling Water

Ingredients:
1/2 cup fresh raspberries
Juice of 2 limes
4 cups sparkling water
Ice cubes

Preparation:
1. In a pitcher, muddle fresh raspberries and lime juice together.
2. Add sparkling water to the pitcher and stir gently.
3. Serve over ice.

Nutritional Value (Approximate):
Calories: 5
Carbohydrates: 1g
Protein: 0g
Fat: 0g

Preparation Time:
5 minutes

Low-FODMAP Cucumber Mint Cooler

Ingredients:
1 cucumber, sliced
810 fresh mint leaves
4 cups cold water
Ice cubes

Preparation:
1. In a pitcher, combine sliced cucumber and fresh mint leaves.
2. Pour cold water over the mixture.
3. Refrigerate for at least 1 hour to infuse flavors.
4. Serve over ice.

Nutritional Value (Approximate):
Calories: 5
Carbohydrates: 1g
Protein: 0g
Fat: 0g

Preparation Time: 5 minutes (+ infusing time)

Low-FODMAP Turmeric Golden Milk

Ingredients:
2 cups unsweetened almond milk
1 teaspoon ground turmeric
1/2 teaspoon ground cinnamon
1/4 teaspoon ground ginger
Pinch of ground black pepper
1 tablespoon maple syrup (optional)

Preparation:
1. In a small saucepan, heat almond milk over medium heat.
2. Whisk in ground turmeric, ground cinnamon, ground ginger, black pepper, and maple syrup (if using).
3. Heat the mixture for 35 minutes until warmed through, but not boiling.
4. Pour into mugs and serve warm.

Nutritional Value (Approximate):
Calories: 40
Carbohydrates: 5g
Protein: 1g
Fat: 2g

Preparation Time: 10 minutes

Low-FODMAP Watermelon Lime Slushie

Ingredients:
4 cups cubed seedless watermelon
Juice of 2 limes
1 tablespoon maple syrup (optional)
Ice cubes

Preparation:
1. Place cubed watermelon in a blender.
2. Add lime juice and maple syrup (if using).
3. Blend until smooth.
4. Add ice cubes and blend again until slushie consistency.
5. Serve immediately.

Nutritional Value (Approximate):
Calories: 60
Carbohydrates: 15g
Protein: 1g
Fat: 0g

Preparation Time: 5 minutes

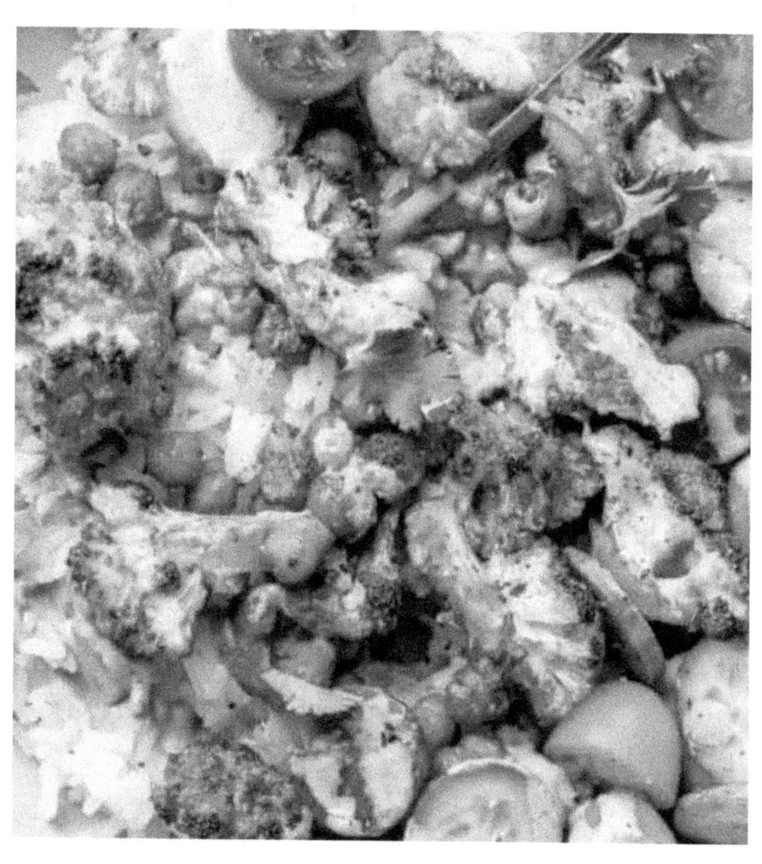

CHAPTER 4

30 DAYS MEAL PLAN

Day 1:

- Breakfast: Banana Berry Smoothie

- Lunch: Quinoa and Vegetable Stir-Fry

- Dinner: Grilled Lemon Herb Chicken

Day 2:

- Breakfast: Low-FODMAP Overnight Oats

- Lunch: Low-FODMAP Tuna Salad

- Dinner: Low-FODMAP Quinoa Stuffed Bell Peppers

Day 3:

- Breakfast: Chia Seed Pudding

- Lunch: Baked Salmon with Roasted Vegetables

- Dinner: Low-FODMAP Beef and Vegetable Stir-Fry

Day 4:

- Breakfast: Spinach and Tomato Frittata

- Lunch: Lentil and Vegetable Soup

- Dinner: Low-FODMAP Pesto Chicken Pasta

Day 5:

- Breakfast: Greek Yogurt Pancakes

- Lunch: Low-FODMAP Chicken Lettuce Wraps

- Dinner: Low-FODMAP Veggie Pizza

Day 6:

- Breakfast: Tofu Scramble Wrap

- Lunch: Low-FODMAP Turkey and Veggie Skewers

- Dinner: Low-FODMAP Ratatouille

Day 7:

- Breakfast: Low-FODMAP Avocado Toast

- Lunch: Eggplant and Tomato Pasta

- Dinner: Low-FODMAP Baked Chicken Thighs

Day 8:

- Breakfast: Low-FODMAP Breakfast Sushi Rolls

- Lunch: Low-FODMAP Chicken and Vegetable Stir-Fry

- Dinner: Low-FODMAP Lemon Garlic Shrimp Pasta

Day 9:

- Breakfast: Low-FODMAP Breakfast Burrito

- Lunch: Low-FODMAP Veggie Quesadilla

- Dinner: Low-FODMAP Quinoa and Black Bean Stuffed Peppers

Day 10:

- Breakfast: Lactose-Free Yogurt Parfait

- Lunch: Low-FODMAP Tofu Lettuce Wraps

- Dinner: Low-FODMAP Stir-Fried Shrimp and Vegetables

Day 11:

- Breakfast: Low-FODMAP Greek Yogurt Parfait

- Lunch: Low-FODMAP Beef and Vegetable Stir-Fry

- Dinner: Low-FODMAP Quinoa and Black Bean Stuffed Peppers

Day 12:

- Breakfast: Low-FODMAP Tofu Scramble Wrap

- Lunch: Low-FODMAP Turkey Wrap

- Dinner: Low-FODMAP Lemon Garlic Shrimp Pasta

Day 13:

- Breakfast: Low-FODMAP Breakfast Hash

- Lunch: Low-FODMAP Chicken Lettuce Wraps

- Dinner: Low-FODMAP Veggie Pizza

Day 14:

- Breakfast: Low-FODMAP Avocado Toast

- Lunch: Lentil and Vegetable Soup

- Dinner: Low-FODMAP Baked Chicken Thighs

Day 15:

- Breakfast: Low-FODMAP Breakfast Sushi Rolls

- Lunch: Low-FODMAP Turkey and Veggie Skewers

- Dinner: Low-FODMAP Ratatouille

Day 16:

- Breakfast: Low-FODMAP Banana Almond Butter Bites

- Lunch: Eggplant and Tomato Pasta

- Dinner: Low-FODMAP Quinoa Stuffed Bell Peppers

Day 17:

- Breakfast: Low-FODMAP Breakfast Burrito

- Lunch: Low-FODMAP Veggie Quesadilla

- Dinner: Low-FODMAP Stir-Fried Shrimp and Vegetables

Day 18:

- Breakfast: Lactose-Free Yogurt Parfait

- Lunch: Low-FODMAP Tofu Lettuce Wraps

- Dinner: Low-FODMAP Baked Salmon with Herbs

Day 19:

- Breakfast: Banana Berry Smoothie

- Lunch: Low-FODMAP Chicken and Vegetable Stir-Fry

- Dinner: Grilled Lemon Herb Chicken

Day 20:

- Breakfast: Low-FODMAP Overnight Oats

- Lunch: Low-FODMAP Tuna Salad

- Dinner: Low-FODMAP Veggie Pizza

Day 21:

- Breakfast: Chia Seed Pudding

- Lunch: Low-FODMAP Turkey Wrap

- Dinner: Low-FODMAP Quinoa Stuffed Bell Peppers
(Recipe #60)

Day 22:

- Breakfast: Low-FODMAP Banana Almond Butter Bites

- Lunch: Low-FODMAP Ratatouille

- Dinner: Low-FODMAP Lemon Garlic Shrimp Pasta

Day 23:

- Breakfast: Low-FODMAP Quinoa Breakfast Bowl

- Lunch: Low-FODMAP Veggie Quesadilla

- Dinner: Low-FODMAP Beef and Vegetable Stir-Fry

Day 24:

- Breakfast: Low-FODMAP Greek-Style Quinoa Bowl

- Lunch: Lentil and Vegetable Soup

- Dinner: Low-FODMAP Quinoa Stuffed Bell Peppers

Day 25:

- Breakfast: Low-FODMAP Breakfast Hash

- Lunch: Low-FODMAP Tofu Lettuce Wraps

- Dinner: Low-FODMAP Baked Chicken Thighs

Day 26:

- Breakfast: Low-FODMAP Breakfast Burrito

- Lunch: Low-FODMAP Turkey Wrap

- Dinner: Low-FODMAP Lemon Garlic Shrimp Pasta

Day 27:

- Breakfast: Banana Berry Smoothie

- Lunch: Low-FODMAP Chicken Lettuce Wraps

- Dinner: Low-FODMAP Veggie Pizza

Day 28:

- Breakfast: Low-FODMAP Overnight Oats

- Lunch: Low-FODMAP Tuna Salad

- Dinner: Low-FODMAP Quinoa Stuffed Bell Peppers

Day 29:

- Breakfast: Lactose-Free Yogurt Parfait

- Lunch: Low-FODMAP Turkey and Veggie Skewers

- Dinner: Grilled Lemon Herb Chicken

Day 30:

- Breakfast: Chia Seed Pudding

- Lunch: Low-FODMAP Stir-Fried Shrimp and Vegetables

- Dinner: Low-FODMAP Baked Salmon with Herbs

CONCLUSION

As we reach the culmination of this low-FODMAP diet cookbook for beginners, it's vital to acknowledge the power food holds in nurturing our wellbeing. The journey through these pages has unveiled the remarkable potential of utilizing food as medicine, not merely for sustenance but as a means to heal and thrive.

Each recipe, guideline, and piece of advice within these pages is an invitation to embark on a transformative journey toward improved health and vitality. Through understanding the intricate relationship between FODMAPs and digestive health, you've gained the tools to make informed dietary choices, paving the way toward a healthier, more balanced lifestyle.

Food isn't solely a source of nutrients; it's a profound healer and sustainer, capable of influencing our physical and mental wellbeing. By consciously choosing low-FODMAP options, one can alleviate digestive discomfort and cultivate a more harmonious relationship between food and the body.

Empowerment through nutrition is the cornerstone of this journey. By taking charge of your dietary habits, you're not only nourishing your body but also reclaiming control over your health. You've learned to listen to your body's cues, personalize your meal plans, and savor the delights of wholesome, nourishing foods.

Remember, this is not just a book; it's an invitation to embrace a lifestyle shift, an empowering journey toward better health. As you continue, stay curious, stay mindful, and relish the transformative power of food in fostering a vibrant and resilient body and mind.

In the end, the true essence lies in the choices you make daily, the conscious decision to prioritize your health and wellbeing through the foods you select. May this journey continue to inspire and guide you on your path to a healthier, more fulfilling life.

Here's to your health, vitality, and the continued embrace of your unique health journey!

MEAL

TRACKER

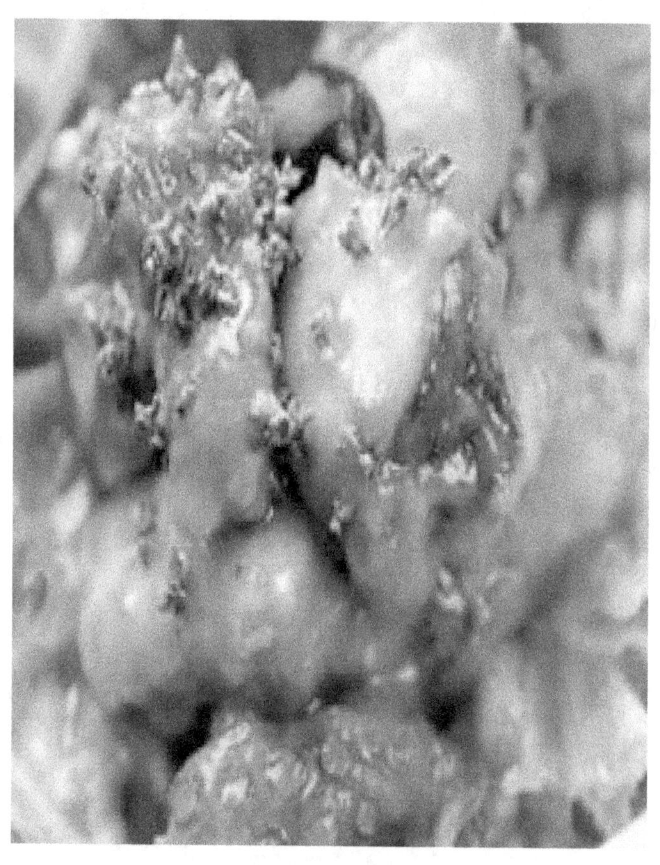

Monday	Breakfast	Lunch	Dinner

Tuesday	Breakfast	Lunch	Dinner

Wednesday	Breakfast	Lunch	Dinner

Thursday	Breakfast	Lunch	Dinner

Friday	Breakfast	Lunch	Dinner

Saturday	Breakfast	Lunch	Dinner

Sunday	Breakfast	Lunch	Dinner

Monday	Breakfast	Lunch	Dinner

Tuesday	Breakfast	Lunch	Dinner

Wednesday	Breakfast	Lunch	Dinner

Thursday	Breakfast	Lunch	Dinner

Friday	Breakfast	Lunch	Dinner

Saturday	Breakfast	Lunch	Dinner

Sunday	Breakfast	Lunch	Dinner

Monday	Breakfast	Lunch	Dinner

Tuesday	Breakfast	Lunch	Dinner

Wednesday	Breakfast	Lunch	Dinner

Thursday	Breakfast	Lunch	Dinner

Friday	Breakfast	Lunch	Dinner

Saturday	Breakfast	Lunch	Dinner

Sunday	Breakfast	Lunch	Dinner

Monday	Breakfast	Lunch	Dinner

Tuesday	Breakfast	Lunch	Dinner

Wednesday	Breakfast	Lunch	Dinner

Thursday	Breakfast	Lunch	Dinner

Friday	Breakfast	Lunch	Dinner

Saturday	Breakfast	Lunch	Dinner

Sunday	Breakfast	Lunch	Dinner

Monday	Breakfast	Lunch	Dinner

Tuesday	Breakfast	Lunch	Dinner

Wednesday	Breakfast	Lunch	Dinner

Thursday	Breakfast	Lunch	Dinner

Friday	Breakfast	Lunch	Dinner

Saturday	Breakfast	Lunch	Dinner

Sunday	Breakfast	Lunch	Dinner

Monday	Breakfast	Lunch	Dinner

Tuesday	Breakfast	Lunch	Dinner

Wednesday	Breakfast	Lunch	Dinner

Thursday	Breakfast	Lunch	Dinner

Friday	Breakfast	Lunch	Dinner

Saturday	Breakfast	Lunch	Dinner

Sunday	Breakfast	Lunch	Dinner

Monday	Breakfast	Lunch	Dinner

Tuesday	Breakfast	Lunch	Dinner

Wednesday	Breakfast	Lunch	Dinner

Thursday	Breakfast	Lunch	Dinner

Friday	Breakfast	Lunch	Dinner

Saturday	Breakfast	Lunch	Dinner

Sunday	Breakfast	Lunch	Dinner

Monday	Breakfast	Lunch	Dinner

Tuesday	Breakfast	Lunch	Dinner

Wednesday	Breakfast	Lunch	Dinner

Thursday	Breakfast	Lunch	Dinner

Friday	Breakfast	Lunch	Dinner

Saturday	Breakfast	Lunch	Dinner

Sunday	Breakfast	Lunch	Dinner

Monday	Breakfast	Lunch	Dinner

Tuesday	Breakfast	Lunch	Dinner

Wednesday	Breakfast	Lunch	Dinner

Thursday	Breakfast	Lunch	Dinner

Friday	Breakfast	Lunch	Dinner

Saturday	Breakfast	Lunch	Dinner

Sunday	Breakfast	Lunch	Dinner

Monday	Breakfast	Lunch	Dinner

Tuesday	Breakfast	Lunch	Dinner

Wednesday	Breakfast	Lunch	Dinner

Thursday	Breakfast	Lunch	Dinner

Friday	Breakfast	Lunch	Dinner

Saturday	Breakfast	Lunch	Dinner

Sunday	Breakfast	Lunch	Dinner